YOUR KNOWLEDGE HAS VALUE

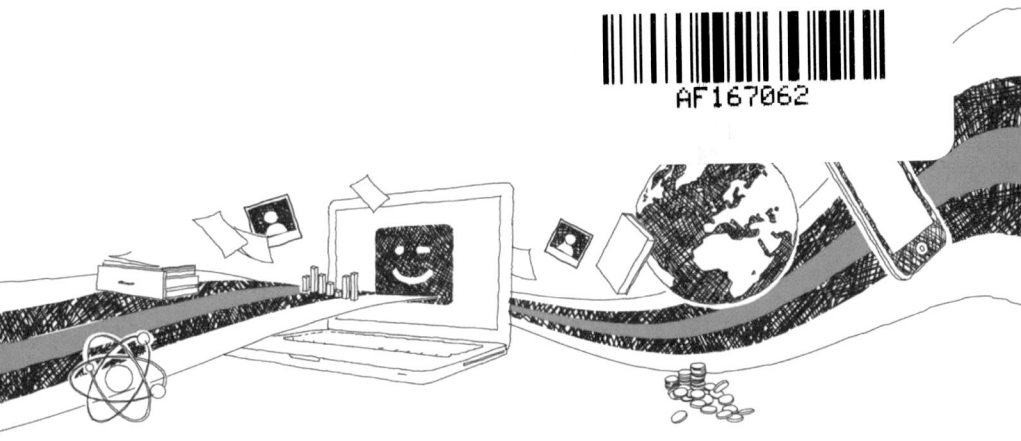
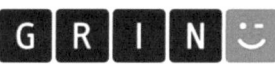

Application of Nanotechnology in Veterinary Medicine

Isayas Asefa

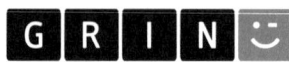

Bibliographic information published by the German National Library:

The German National Library lists this publication in the National Bibliography; detailed bibliographic data are available on the Internet at http://dnb.dnb.de.

ISBN: 9783346643131
This book is also available as an ebook.

© GRIN Publishing GmbH
Nymphenburger Straße 86
80636 München

Print and binding: Books on Demand GmbH, Norderstedt, Germany
Printed on acid-free paper from responsible sources.

GRIN web shop: https://www.grin.com/document/1194974

Review on Application of Nano Technology in Veterinary Medicine

Isayas Asefa

Wolaita Sodo University, School of Veterinary Medicine, DVM Student, Wolaita Sodo, Ethiopia.

Abstract

Nanotechnology is research and technology development at the atomic, molecular and macromolecular levels at the scale of approximately 1 - 100 nanometer range, to provide a fundamental understanding of phenomena and materials at the nano scale and to create and use structures, devices and systems that have novel properties and functions because of their small and/or intermediate size. Nanotechnology has the potential to solve many more puzzles related to animal health, products and breeding. The applications of nanotechnology become the proving ground for untried and more controversial techniques from Nano capsule vaccines to sex selection in breeding. There are numerous applications of nanotechnology in veterinary medicine including disease diagnosis, treatment, drug delivery, animal breeding and improving and boosting animal origin food product. It is swiftly changing the diagnosis and treatment patterns at faster and low cost in less time duration. In general, the application with nanotechnology in the field of veterinary medicine was very broad and further investigations are very quartile for effective utilization of the technology in the practical life in making sustainable demand and supply system with human need in advancing world.

Keywords: *Diagnosis, nanomaterials, nanotechnology, treatment.*

Inhalt

1. INTRODUCTION 3

2. DEFINITION OF NANOTECHNOLOGY 3

    2.1. Application of Nanotechnology in disease diagnosis 4

    2.2. Application of Nanotechnology in drug delivery system and Treatments 6

    2.3. Antimicrobials Nanoparticles in veterinary medicine 8

    2.4. Nano vaccine and vaccine adjuvant 9

    2.5. Application of nanotechnology in animal breeding 9

    2.6. Application of nanotechnology in animal and chicken product 10

3. CONCLUSION AND RECOMMENDATION 12

4. REFERENCES 13

1. INTRODUCTION

Nanotechnology is an exciting and rapidly emerging technology allowing us to work at the molecular level, often atom by atom, to create and manipulate tools, materials and functional structures that have nanometer dimensions. Nature has been performing 'Nano technological feats' for millions of years. Through the arrangement of atoms and molecules, biological systems combine wet chemistry and electro-chemistry in a single living system. It used within the body, within the cells for diagnosing and treatment of diseases. It has the potential to have greats impact on diagnosis and treatment of animals. Unique size dependent properties of nanoparticles have numerous diagnostic applications such as diagnostic biosensors, imaging nanoprobes for magnetic resonance imaging contrast agents (Prabaharan *et al.*, 2010). Using nanotechnology multifunctional nanomaterial's can be designed to image a specific organ, target tissue, access deep molecular targets and provide drugs at controlled release. Great advances have been and are being made in nanobiochip materials, nanoscale biomimetic materials, nanomotors, nanocomposite materials, interface biomaterials and nanobiosensors with enormous prospect in veterinary medicine application (Tiwari *etal.* 2011).

It is a research and development aimed at understanding and working with seeing, measuring and manipulating at the atomic, molecular and supramolecular levels. This correlates to length scales of roughly 1 to 100 nanometers. At this scale, the physical, chemical and biological properties of materials differ fundamentally and often unexpectedly integrated sensing, monitoring and controlling system could detect the presence of disease and notify the farmer and veterinarian to activate a targeted treatment delivery system This is possible with nanotechnology and could permit a wide range of advances in the field of agriculture, animal and veterinary sciences such as conversion of agricultural and food wastes to energy and other useful by-products through enzymatic nanobioprocessing, development in reproductive sciences, breeding managements, disease prevention and treatment in animals and public health (Patil *et al* .,2004). Applications of nanotechnology and nanoparticles in food, animal breeding and animal productivity such as in meat production, milk production are emerging rapidly. It used to create materials and change structure, enhanced quality and texture of foodstuffs at the molecular level. This technology has a major impact on production, processing, transportation, storage, traceability, safety and security of food (Otles and Yalcin, 2008).

Therefore, the objective of this seminar paper is to review the application of nanotechnology on smart drug delivery system, in animal disease treatment and diagnosis, animal breeding and reproduction and also chicken product.

2. DEFINITION OF NANOTECHNOLOGY

The term "Nanotechnology"was frist applied in 1970s and was used to production technology at ultrafine dimensions, hence the use of the Greek word ''nano''-meaning Dwarf. According to the published document of International Organization for Standardization (IOS), nanotechnology is defined as a scientific knowledge application for matter's manipulation and control in Nano metric scale (Troncarelli *et al.*, 2008).

3

The most widely use definition of nanotechnology is provided by the United States Government's National Nanotechnology Initiative. According to the researchers, nanotechnology is defined as: "Research and technology development at the atomic, molecular and macromolecular levels at the scale of approximately 1 - 100 nanometer range, to provide a fundamental understanding of phenomena and materials at the nanoscale and to create and use structures, devices and systems that have novel properties and functions because of their small and/or intermediate size (Feneque, 2003).

The generic term of 'nano-object' as defined by the European union Commission recommendation on a code of conduct for responsible nanosciences and nanotechnologies research will include all nanomaterial's, nanostructured materials, nanoparticles and their aggregation at the nanoscale, nano-systems, and nanoproducts (Brussels, 2008).

2.1. Application of Nanotechnology in disease diagnosis

Nanotechnology has the potential to provide cheaper, fast and precise diagnostic tools. These days, nanomaterials are playing a key role in imaging and monitoring and hence earlier detection of disease. Better diagnosis has a positive effect in the cost of animal health care. Bio nanomaterial based research has emerged as a new exciting field and DNA, RNA and peptides are considered as important bionanomaterials for the fundamental development in life sciences. The nanomaterial's such as quantum dots, nano shells, carbon nanotubes can be synthesized and functionalized which may couple with the imaging sources and accompany the molecule with ultrasound, magnetic resonance, X-rays techniques to diagnose the targeted organ effectively (Loukanov *et al.*, 2012).

2.1.1. Nano chips

Earlier and rapid detection of diseases causing pathogens was done by wide range of assays like enzyme immunosorbent assay, western blot assay, polymerase chain reaction, neutralization, agar-gel immunodiffusion (Hirsch *et al.*, 2003).
Nano chips have diverse range of applications ranging from recognizing genes, guiding drug delivery to monitoring body functions and perceive life science and chemical pathogens. Nanochips are also applied for identification of certain diseases like cystic fibrosis and scanning of DNA for signs of predispositions of other ailments (Wei *et al.*, 2010).
Nanochips have been employed to detect gene mutations responsible for monogenic disorders that help to determine etiology of complex diseases including heart disease, diabetes and neuro psychiatric traits. Recently, researchers developed silver sputtered nanochip that mimic the connectivity between neurons in the brain (Chang et *al.*, 2010).

2.1.2. Nano sensors

Nano sensors are miniature devices that can diagnose samples which use biological material or tissue based on bio recognition element which is immobilized on the surface of physicochemical transducer. Applications of nanosensors open great prospectives ranging from whole body monitoring to diagnosing various diseases due to their unprecedented sensitivity. Majorly, nano sensors are based on two detection principles catalytic and affinity sensing. Catalytic sensors utilize enzymes, cells, tissues and microorganisms as the recognition agent. Affinity sensors are those which utilize whole antibodies, antibody fragments, nucleic acid, receptors, lectins, phages, novel engineered scaffold derived bonding proteins, molecular imprinted polymers, plastic antibodies and synthetic protein binding agents as the recognition agent (Akkoyun et al., 2000).

Nanosensors have major role in veterinary sciences, they use very small amount of a chemical contaminant, virus or bacteria which is helpful for agriculture and food systems that in return improves the feedstock (Scott, 2005).

2.1.3. Liposomes

Vesicles composed of a lipid bilayer surrounding a hollow core; they can be composed of natural phospholipids or other surfactants and Drugs or other molecules can be loaded for delivery to tumors or other disease sites; Liposome's can carry both hydrophobic and hydrophilic drugs and molecules to a target site (Mcmillan etal., 2011). The major types of liposomes are the multilamellar vesicle, the small unilamellar and large unilamellar vesicles, and the cochleate vesicle. Owing to the diversity of their structures and compositions, liposomes have become versatile tools in clinical applications in cancer treatment (imaging and therapy)(Wang etal., 2008). Flexibility of liposome construction allows incorporation of imaging agents into either the bilayer or interior, making them effective carriers for intensification of contrast in magnetic resonance imaging and computed tomography (Zheng etal., 2006).

Liposomes are small artificial vesicles of spherical shape composed of single or multiple concentric bilayers, size ranging from 50-500 nm. Liposomes play a key role in diagnosis as they can be used as carriers for radioisotopes and contrast agents. Liposome can be used in blood pool or perfusion and lymphatic imaging based on contrast enhancement. The potential of paramagnetic liposome in blood pool, lymphatic and perfusion imaging was proven by various *ex vivo* and *in vivo* animal studies (Suga et al., 2001).

2.1.4. Quantum dots

Quantum dots are semiconductor nanocrystals having unique properties like high level of photostablility, tunable optical properties, single-wavelength excitation and size-tunable emission. Due to their extremely small size (around 10 nm in diameter), they are used as fluorescent probes for bio molecular and cellular imaging (Azzay et al., 2006).). A quantum dot enables high sensitive detection of analytes at low concentrations due to their similar quantum efficiencies. Diseases involving large number of genes and proteins can be detected by multicolor quantum dot probe that helps in imaging and tracking multiple molecular targets simultaneously (Samia et al., 2003). Quantum dots offer a multipurpose nanoscale framework for defining and constructing versatile nanoparticles that can be utilized to carry out both functions, in imaging and treatment (Misra etal., 2010) . Quantum dots offer major advantages over radioactive tags or fluorospheres like fluorescin or cyanine dyes in terms of longevity due to their stability and resistance to photo bleaching(Cuenca etal., 2006).

2.1.5. Magnetic nanoparticles

Magnetic nanoparticles are finding increasing applications in the areas of diagnostic and therapeutic because of the advantageous properties associated with the lesser dipoledipole interactions, lower sedimentation rates, facilitation in tissue diffusion, high magnetization so as to be controlled by external magnetic fields and to reach the targeted pathologic tissue and their small size that make them available for circulation through the capillary systems of organs and tissues (Sobik et al.,2011). Magnetic nanoparticles have been widely used in the early diagnosis of diseases. They are especially important for some fatal diseases such as cancer. Some magnetic nanoparticles like iron oxide nanoparticles have been used in perfusion imaging for *in-vivo* characterization of tumors (Strijkers et al., 2005). Magnetic nanoparticles show effective results in animal body as they can easily move in liquid medium and thus can be excited magnetically or detected inside nonmagnetic tissue (Zhao *etal*., 2011).

2.2. Application of Nanotechnology in drug delivery system and Treatments

2.2.1. Application of Nanotechnology in drug delivery systems

Considering the Pharmacology area, nanotechnology allows the development of new products and also the possibility to rework conventional substances in order to obtain better efficacy results, by loading drugs into nanoparticles through physical encapsulation, adsorption, or chemical conjugation, the pharmacokinetics and therapeutic index of the drugs can be significantly improved in contrast to the free drug counterparts. Drug-loaded nanoparticles can enter host cells through endocytosis and then release drug payloads to treat microbes-induced intracellular infections (Zhang *et al*., 2010).

Nanoparticle-based drug delivery provides many advantages, such as enhancing drug-therapeutic efficiency and pharmacological characteristics. The utility of nanoparticles in improving pharmacokinetics, reducing unwanted side effects, and improving delivery to disease sites has been demonstrated for a number of nanodrug delivery systems (Suh *et al*., 2009). For example, nanoparticles improve the solubility of poorly water-soluble drugs, modify pharmacokinetics, increase drug half-life by reducing immunogenicity, increase specificity towards the target cell or tissue (therefore Reducing side effects), improve bioavailability, diminish drug metabolism and enable a more controllable release of therapeutic compounds and the delivery of two or more drugs simultaneously for combination therapy (Allen and Cullis, 2004).

Generally, the practical consequences of a pharmaceutical nanostructure substance are providing a rational use of the active ingredient, considering that both the number of doses and the concentration of the drug may be reduced during the treatment and "Renewing" of old pharmaceutical bases which were continued used and also prolonging the systemic circulation lifetime of drug. Releasing drugs at a sustained and controlled manner, preferentially delivering drugs to the tissues and cells of interest, delivering multiple therapeutic agents to the same cells for combination therapy (Peer *et al*., 2007). Providing new perspectives of administration routes for medicines and vaccines and also reducing stress and toxicity for drug administration, collateral effects of conventional pharmaceutical actives. Providing the use of new molecules and actives in animal therapeutic and producing low (or none) residues in animal products, resulting in no withdrawal needed (Zhag *et al*., 2008).

2.2.2. Application of Nanotechnology in Treatment of disease

The effective delivery of therapeutic molecules has been a major barrier to obtain targeted response against the disease agent. Many drugs are effective in treating diseases but most of them also have certain limitations with regard to toxicity, poor aqueous solubility and cell impermeability. The drawbacks discussed above can be solved by Nanomedicine. Nano medicine has the potential to solve unique biological challenges. New drugs and new delivery systems both come under "Nanomedicine" umbrella. Therapeutic and diagnostic agents are at the forefront projects of Nanomedicine and research is focused on rational delivery and targeting of pharmaceuticals in animals (Desai *et al.*, 1997).

Nano pharmaceuticals, the most promising and productive area of nanotechnology application in animal treatment involves nanoparticles and hence they are available for broad range of biological targets owing to their small size and higher mobility. Nano pharmaceuticals engross encapsulating the material to generate nanoparticle which thereby improves solubility, diffusion and degradation characteristics of the encapsulated material and, nanomaterials that can carry drugs to the targeted site (Si *et al.*, 2007).

2.2.3. Polymeric Nanoparticles

Strategies for controlled drug-delivery have made a considerable progress in the field of veterinary medicine where polymeric nanoparticles play a key role. They deliver drugs for long periods, increasing the drug efficacy, maximizing the patient compliance thereby enhancing the ability to use highly toxic, poorly soluble or relatively unstable drugs. They are used for the development of highly selective and efficient therapeutic and diagnostic modalities (Frietas, 1998). Polymeric nanoparticles can circulate freely in the body and penetrate tissues by means of mechanisms such as endocytosis(Gao *etal.*,2004). Polymeric nanoparticles are structurally stable and can be synthesized with a sharper size distribution. Polymeric nanoparticles are usually coated with nonionic surfactants in order to reduce immunological interactions as well as intermolecular interactions between the surface of chemical group polymeric nanoparticles (Agnieszka *etal.*, 2012).

2.2.4. Carbon nanotubes

Carbon nanotubes have potential therapeutic applications in the field of drug delivery. They can be functionalized by various biomolecules such as bioactive peptides, proteins, nucleic acids and drugs, and are used to deliver their cargos to cells and organs (Tiwari and Dhakate, 2009). Though the mechanism of cell penetration is not fully understood, it is suggested that their needle-like shape enables them to penetrate cellular membranes and enter into intracellular content without significant damage to the cell(Cai *etal.*, 2005).

2.2.5. Nanoshells

Nanoshells are concentric particles in which one material is coated with a thin layer of another material by various synthesis methods. Nanoshells are currently being used in cancer chemotherapy and still more applications are conceived in the treatment of diseases . Gold nanoshells destroy the cancer completely. They can also be used to immobilize cells or viruses, to trap and embed small and macromolecules on surfaces (Kumar, 2007).

2.2.6. Dendrimers

Dendrimers have a range of applications from drug delivery to drug diagnosis. It considered as potential drug carriers for treatment of diseases with the capability to provide a sustained release along with reduced side effect and rapid pharmacological response with improved efficacy. Dendrimers are effectively used in drug delivery as they deliver a drug at controlled rate by chemically modifying them either by fine tuning of hydrolytic release conditions and the selective leakage of drug molecules on the basis of their size or shape or by pH-sensitive materials (Jansen *et al.*, 1995). Dendrimers are defined as highly ordered and regularly branched globular macromolecules produced by stepwise iterative approaches (Svenson and Tomalia, 2006). The drug may be encapsulated in the internal structure of dendrimers or it can be chemically attached or physically adsorbed on dendrimers surface (Menjoge et al.,2010).

2.3. Antimicrobials Nanoparticles in veterinary medicine

The field of veterinarian sciences stands to gain with nanotechnology diagnostic tools (nanoprobes) that can be used in vitro and on living animals,targeted delivery of medications, therapeutic nanomaterial's, vaccine antigen vectors, in vivo imagery, or traceability of products of animal origin. An important increase of scientific researches for nanostructured products development in the last years has been verified in Veterinary Medicine, especially using antimicrobials actives. Conventional synthetic and natural antimicrobial substances are being tested, and have shown excellent results against multi-resistant microorganisms and bacteria strains that are normally hard to eliminate by using the conventional treatment, like *Brucella abortus, Mycobacterium bovis, Staphylococcus aureus, Salmonella, Ehrlichia, Ana plasma; Rhodococcus equi*, etc. (Mcmillan *et al.*, 2011).

2.3.1. Invitro studies –conventional antimicrobials

Nanostructured *streptomycin* and *doxycyclin*e were tested against *Brucella melitensis strains*, and the efficacy results of nanoparticles were better than the conventional antimicrobials (Seleem *etal.*, 2009). This specific pathogen usually stays inside animal's macrophages, and its pharmacological control is very hard. In this *in vitro* study, both antimicrobial actives were encapsulated in anfihilicpolymer's, allowing the nanoparticles to reach the interior of murine macrophages. When tested *in vivo* (in infected marine's), the nanostructured formulation determined reduction of the number of colony-forming unities and also with a better efficacy compared to the conventional formulation. *Escherichia coli* and *Salmonella typhi* bacteria are two common pollutants and they are developing resistance to the most used bactericide. New biocide materials are being tested. Thus, gold nanoparticles are proposed to inhibit the growth of these two microorganisms. Gold nanoparticles dispersed on zeolites eliminate *Escherichia coli* and *Salmonella typhi* colonies at short time (Lima *et al.*, 2013).

2.3.2. Invitro studies with Ag nanoparticles

The antimicrobial effects of silver ion or salts are well known, and the silver nanoparticles show efficient antimicrobial property compared to other salts. The Ag nanostructures are most effective on *E. coli, yeast S. aureus, Klebsiella* and *Pseudomonas*. These nanoparticles preferably attack the respiratory chain and cell division, finally leading to cell death. Ag nanoparticles can be used as effective growth inhibitors in various microorganisms, making them applicable to diverse medical devices and antimicrobial control systems. The scanning transmission electron microscopy confirms the presence of silver in the cell membrane and inside bacteria (Rajasokkapan, 2013).

2.3.3. In vitro studies of nanoparticles composed by natural antimicrobial actives

The antimicrobial activity and bactericide effect of propolis against a wide range of bacteria, fungi, yeasts and viruses have been investigated since the late 1940s and it showed variable activity against different microorganisms. The alcoholic extracts of propolis inhibited the growth of various bacteria, including strains of streptococci and Bacillus. The inhibition of bacterial RNA polymerase by the components of propolis is probably due to the loss of their ability to bind to DNA (Hepazi, 2013).

2.4. Nano vaccine and vaccine adjuvant

Vaccination is one of the important methods of prevention of disease in advance by developing antibody against the particular pathogen. Nanoparticles used as vaccine carriers and adjuvants. Synthetic oligodeoxynucleotides and antigens in biodegradable nanospheres used for immunization .A better immune response seem to be obtained with biodegradable nanospheres vaccines produced by conventional methods. These new perspectives for vaccines development are contributing with better efficacy and safety results, both in pets and livestock animals (Akagi *et al.*, 2012).

Liposomal vaccines can be made by associating microbes, soluble antigens, and cytokine. Liposomes as vaccine adjuvant, liposomes have been firmly established as immunoadjuvants (enhancers of the immunological response), potentiating both cell mediated and humoral immunity. Liposomal immune adjuvants act by slowly releasing encapsulated antigen on intramuscular injection and also by passively accumulating within regional lymph nodes (Gregoriadis, 1995).

Adjuvants are agents added to a vaccine to augment immune responses toward antigens. A number of studies describe the use of nanoparticles as adjuvant. Immunization of animals with both complete antigens and haptens (small molecules that can elicit an immune response only when attached to a large carrier such as a nanoparticle or a protein) conjugated to the surface of colloidal gold particles generated higher levels of specific antibodies than immunization of the same antigens with classical adjuvants. Furthermore, the amount of antigen required to achieve a high antibody response was an order of magnitude lower than for immunization with Freund's adjuvant (Andreev, 2000).

2.5. Application of nanotechnology in animal breeding

Nanotechnology has begun to blossom in the field of reproduction and fertility (Verma *etal.*, 2012). In this way, the aims of these nanotechnology-based investigations related to animal reproduction are characterize the nanoscale features of gamete cells using atomic force microscopy and related scanning probe microscopy techniques(Carvalho *etal.*, 2013). Management of breeding is an expensive and time-consuming problem for canine, dairy and swine farmers. One solution that is currently being studied is a nanotube implanted under the skin to provide real time measurement of changes in the level of estradiol in the blood. The nanotubes are used as a means of tracking oestrus in animal because these tubes have the capacity to bind and detect the estradiol antibody at the time of oestrus by near infrared fluorescence. The signal from this sensor will be incorporated as a part of a central monitoring and control system to actual breeding (O'Connell *et al.*, 2002). The goal of all these innovative efforts is not just to be able to characterize and manipulate the matter on nanoscale, but also develop products and processes with economic, social and environmental value added with emphasis on the development of solutions to animal reproduction challenges(Weibel *etal.*, 2014).

2.6. Application of nanotechnology in animal and chicken product

2.6.1. Meat production/industry sector (nanomeat)

Nanotechnology study individual nanoparticles and their unique application for meat industry ranging from meat design, achieving food security, meat safety, overcoming food allergies, eliminating pesticide use, meat packaging, restoring meat damage and sensory evaluation to processes such as filtration, separation, encapsulation etc. (Mallika *et al.*, 2005). One of the more futuristic applications of nanotechnology lies in the production of "interactive" poultry meat that changecolour, flavour or nutrients depending on diner's taste or health (Marquez, 2004). There were many methods to improve livestock meat products by nanotechnology. Encapsulation system, at present spray drying, melts extrusion, co-acervation, coating with fat and sprays chilling are commonly employed encapsulation techniques. The encapsulation system using nanotechnology has numerous benefits as detailed below (Raj Kumar *et al.*, 2006).

Taste masking, head-triggered release consecutive delivery of multiple active ingredients, change in flavor character and long lasting organoleptic perception of nanotechnologies ranging from the actual to the speculative promise a variety of ways to create real meat without killing animals. On top of this, add the promise that genetic engineering could produce cells that have a variety of new qualities that would make meat eve healthier and tastier: higher protein, lower fat, high omega 3 acid levels or other healthful concoctions (Kolata, 2006).

Some of the researchers in this field, for instance, are so committed to the development of cultured meat—largely out organizations to pursue the technology. For example, New Harvest is a ''non-profit research organization working to develop new meat substitutes, including cultured meat—meat produced in vitro, in a cell culture, rather than from an animal. Cultured meat has the potential to make eating animals unnecessary, even while satisfying all the nutritional and hedonic requirements of meat eaters. It also has the potential to greatly reduce animal suffering (Hopkins and Dacey, 2008).

2.6.2. Milk production/industry sector (nanomilk)

Nanotechnology is a new technological tool in modern raw milk production and pasteurization, recent and ongoing advances in biomedical technology will assist in advancing our understanding of disease prevention and health promotion, as well as medical diagnostics and therapeutics (Ross *et al.*, 2004).
Recent developments of nanotechnological tools begins to bring sophisticated Polymerase Chain Reaction (PCR) methods, cantilever systems, various microarray systems, new biosensors, etc. This substantiates an intensified research in new solid on-line/at line methods, which can measure critical points throughout the milk production chain (e.g., feed, cow, raw milk, milk tank, throughout the processing chain, during storage and distribution with regard to pathogens, indicator organisms of contamination, antibiotics, toxins, chemical contaminants, and allergens). These support the development of hazard analysis critical control points (HACCP)-based quality management systems. Development of mentioned HACCP-based quality management systems as well as shelf-

life prediction systems also calls for development of sophisticated modeling of growth and decline of pathogens, spoilers and contaminants in the milk and dairy products (Andersen, 2007).

Liposomes micelles used to encapsulate both water and lipid soluble compounds. The dissolution of fat-soluble nutrients in water-based drinks is one of the key applications of liposomes. Examples of current research into the use of liposome technology in food are the encapsulation of enzymes, lactic acid bacteria extracts and/or antimicrobials for accelerated cheese ripening. Liposome technology can be used potentially to target specific sites within a food product for enzymatic degradation (Taylor *et al.*, 2005).

2.6.3. Egg production/industry sector (nanoegg)

Poultry meat and eggs are often the source food borne pathogens, like salmonella. Early detection of food borne pathogenic bacteria is critical to prevent disease outbreaks and preserve public health. Now, a novel nanotechnology-based biosensor is showing great potential for forborne pathogenic bacteria detection with high accuracy (Park, 2008).

Nanotechnology has to supply cholesterol free eggs, yolkless or reduced yolk eggs which can be the high value protein source, immune eggs which can supply the predetermined antibodies and therapeutic eggs with supply the predetermined physiological factors for treatment purposes. The tools and techniques currently with us will not give the solution for these challenges. They can only be meeting out by the emerging nanotechnology, which deals not merely at the molecular level but at the atomic level (Kannaki and Verma, 2006).

3. CONCLUSION AND RECOMMENDATION

Nanotechnology has emerged as one of the most innovative technologies and has potential to provide fast and precise drug delivery system, diagnostic nanomaterial tools and therapeuatic nanoparticle and nanomedicine (nanodrug). These nanomaterials are playing a key role in diseases diagnosis, treatment, drug delivery, animal nutrition, breeding, reproductions and values additions to animals' product. Nanoparticles also play great role in disease diagnosis at molecular levels as well as at a single cell by using different nanomaterials.

Also, nanotechnology in livestock product, such as in meat and milk, has key role. In the future it provides new products and new processes, with the goal of enhancing the performance of the product, prolonging the product shelf life and freshness, and improving the Safety and quality of animal origin food.

Based on the above conclusion the following recommendations are forwarded:

- Continuous research should be conducted on nanotechnology, particularly on nanobiotechnology in animal science and veterinary medicine in order to increase production of low fat and low cholesterol animal products.
- More advanced research should be conducted on nanoparticle, nanomaterial and nanomedicine to improve effective diagnosis and treatment of animal diseases.
- Ethiopian governments should give a great attention to nanotechnology and they must support the Scientists and researchers who investigate nanotechnology.

4. REFERENCES

Agnieszka, Z., Wilczewska1, Niemirowicz, K,Markiewicz1K.H, Car.H. (2012): Nanoparticles as drug delivery systems. *Pharmacological Reports*, **64**: 1020-1037.

Akagi, T., Baba, M., and Akashi, M. (2012): Biodegradable nanoparticles as vaccine adjuvant and delivery systems: regulation of immune responses by nanoparticle-based vaccine. *Advanced Polymer Science*, **247**: 31–64.

Akkoyun, A., Kohen, V.F., and Bilitewski, U. (2000): Detection of sulphamethazine with an optical biosensor and anti-idiotypic antibodies. *Sensory Actuators Biology*, **70**:12. DOI: http://dx.doi.org/10.1016/S0925-4005 (00)00547-5.

Allen, T.M., and Cullis, P.R. (2004): Drug delivery systems: entering the mainstream. *Science directory*, **30** (3):1818-1822.

Andersen, H.J., (2007): The issue raw milk quality from the point of view of a major dairy industry. *Journal of Animal Feed Science*, **16**:240-254.

Andreev, S.M., (2000): An immunogenic and allergenic property of fullerene conjugates with amino acid and proteins. *Doklady Biochemistry*. **370**: 4–7.

Azzazy, E.M., Hassan, M.H., and Kazmierczak, C. S. (2006): Quantum Dot Study Opens Door to New Clinical Cancer Tools. *Journal of Clinical Chemistry*, **52**(7):1238. DOI: 10.1373/clinchem.2006.066654.

Banson, P., (2008): Nanotechnology biosensor to detect *Salmonella*.2008. http://www.scopemed.org/mnstemps/2/2-129191428 http://www.worldpoultry. Accessed on march, 29th ,2017.

Brussels, A. (2008): Commission recommendation of 07/02/2008 on a Code of Conduct for Responsible Nanosciences and Nanotechnologies Research. Prossed in the WHO, annual conference, Belgium, Brussels.

Cai D, Mataraza JM, Qin ZH, Huang Z, Huang J,(2005) : Highly efficient molecular delivery into mammalian cells using carbon nanotube spearing. *Naturals Methods* **2**: 449-454.

Carvalho, J.O., L.P. Silva, R. Sartori and A.N. Dode, (2013): Nanoscale differences in the shape and size of X and Y chromosome-bearing bovine sperm heads assessed by atomic force microscopy. PLOS ONE (8[th]Eds), **5**:87-93

Chang, T.E., Bhadviya, I., B.B., Lu W., and Mazumder, P. (2010): Nanoscale memristor device as synapse in neuromorphic systems, *Nanotechnology Letters*, **10** (4): 1297. DOI: 10.1021/nl904029h.

Cuenca, AG., Jiang H., Hochwald SN, Delano M., Cance WG. (2006):Emerging implications of nanotechnology on cancer diagnostics and therapeutics. *Cancer*, **107**: 459-466.

Desai, M.P., and Labhasetwar, V., Walter, E., Levy, R.J., and Amidon, G.L. (1997): The mechanism of uptake of biodegradable micro particles in Caco-2 cells is size dependent.*Pharmaceutical Research,* **14**: *1568.* DOI:10.1023/a:1012126301290

Fenque, J., (2013): Brief introduction to the Veterinary applications ofNanotechnology: www.Nanotech-now.com/JoseFeneque/VeterinaryApplicaion .Accessed March 29, 2017.

Frietas, R.A., (1998): Natural Polymer Drug Delivery Systems: Nanoparticles, Plants, and Algae. *Artificial Cells Blood Substitution Immobilization Biotechnology*, **26**: 411. DOI: 10.4103/0972-124X.44088.

Gao, X., Y. Cui, R.M. Levenson, W.K. Chung and S. Nie, (2004):Invivo cancer targeting and imaging with semiconductor quantum dots. *Nature Biotechnology*,**22**: 969-76.

Gregoriadis, G., (1995): Engineering liposome's for drug delivery: progress and problems. *Trends in biotechnology,* **13***:*527-537.

Hegazi, A.G., (2013): Propolis an overview. *Journal of basic medical science.*Available in www.apinetla.com.ar/congreso/c05 Accessed on March, 29th, 2017.

Hirsch, L.R., (2003). A whole blood immunoassay using gold nanoshells. *Analytical Chemistry* , **75** (10): 2377- 2381. http://www.nytimes.com/2006/03/27/health/27pig.html?ex=1168318800& en5706ef70a33c702&ei=5070. Accessed March, 29th, 2017.

Jansen, J.F., Meijer, A, E.W., Berg, E.M.M., and Brabandar-Vanden. J. *(*1995): Molecular modeling of dendrimers for nanoscale application. *American Chemical society,* **177**: 4417. DOI: 10.1021/ja00120a032.

Kannaki, T.R., and P.C. Verma, (2006): The challenges of 2020 and the role of nanotechnology in poultry research. Proceedings of the National Seminar on Poultry Research Priorities to. *Centre of Avian Research Institute*(Indian council of agricultural research).Izatnagar-243:122 (U.P) .India.

Kolata, G. (2006). Cloning may lead to healthier pork. *journal of agriculture,* New York Times, March 27.Retrived from March 29, 2017.

Kumar, C., (2007): Wiley VCH Verlag GmbH & Co. KGaA, Weinheim, 5: Nanoscale device for veterinary Technology: *trends and future prospective,* **5:**

Lima, E., Guerra, R., Laraand, V., Guzmán, A. (2013): Gold nanoparticles as efficient antimicrobial agents for *Escherichia coli* and *Salmonella typhi. Chemistry of Central Journal,* 7: 11.

Loukanov, A.R., Emin, S., Tiwari A., Mishra, A. K., Kobayashi, H., and Turner A. (2012): In *Intelligent Nanomaterials*, Wiley-Scrivener Publishing (2nd edition), LLC, USA, 649-664. ISBN 978-04-709387-99.

Mallika, C., Pandey, M.C., Radhakrishna, K., and Bawa, A.S. (2005): Nano-Technology: Applications in Food Industry. *Indian Food Industry,* **24***:* 19-21.

Marquez, M., (2004): Nanotechnology to Play Important and Prominent Role in Food Safety http://www.azonano.com/details.asp?ArticleID=858matroncarelli@yahoo. comAccessed March 29, 2017.

McMillan, J., Batrakova, E., and Gendelmnh, E. (2011): Cell Delivery of Therapeutic Nanoparticles. *Proceeding in Molecular Biology and Translational Science,* **104**:563-601.

Menjoge, A.R, Kannan, R.M., Tomalia, D.A. (2010): Dendrimer based drug and imaging conjugates: design considerations for nanomedical applications. *Drug Discovery Today*, **15**:171–187.

Misra, R., Acharya, S., Sahoo, SK . (2010) : Cancer nanotechnology:application of nanotechnology in cancer therapy. *Drug Discov Today,* **15**:842-850

Monerris, M.J., F.J. Arévalo, H. Fernández, M.A. Zon and P.G. Molina. (2012): Integrated electrochemical immunosensor with gold nanoparticles for the determination of progesterone. *Sensory Actuators Biochemistry*, **166**(6):586-592.

Oconnell, M.J., Bachilo, S.M., Huffaman, C.B., Moore, V.C., Strano, M.S., Haroz, E.H., Rialon, K.L., Boul, P.J., Kittrell, C., Hauge, R.H., Weisman, R.B., and Smalley R.E. (2002): Band gap fluorescence from individual single walled carbon nanotubes. *Science,* **297**:593- 596.

Park, H., Han, H. (2002): Production and characterization of biodegradable povidine-iodine as intrammary disinfectant. *Journal VeterinarySciences,* **64** (8):739-741.

Pathak, P.A., (2008):Application of magnetic nanoparticles. *Nanomedicine and Nanobiotechnology*, **1**:84. DOI: 10.1002/wnan.17

Patil, S.S., K, B. Kore and Puneet, Kumar. (2004): Nanotechnology and its applications in Veterinary and Animal Science. *Veterinary World*, **2** (12): 475-477.

Patrick, D.H., and Austin, D. (2008): Vegetarian Meat: Could Technology Save Animals and Satisfy Meat Eaters. *Journals of Agriculture and Environmental Ethics,* **21**: 579–596.

Peer, D., Karp, J. M., Hong, S., Farokhzad, O. C., Margalit, R. and Langer, R. (2007): Nanocarriers as an emerging platform for cancer therapy. *Nature of Nanotechnology*, **2**:751- 760.

Prabaharan, M., Jayakumar, R., and Tiwari, A. (2010)**:** In Recent Developments in Bio-Nanocomposites for Biomedical Applications; Tiwari, A. (4th edition) Nova

Science Publishers: New York, USA, 17-40 ISBN: 978-1-61761-008-0. DOI: 10.1007/s11259-007-0080-x.

Rajasokkapan, S., (2013): Applications of Nanotechnology in Veterinary Science. Available in: http://www.slideshare.net/sokkappan/nanotechnology-in-veterinary medicine. Accessed in March 29, 2017.

Rajkumar, R.S., Kandeepan, G., Prejit and Susitha, R. (2006): Applications of Nano-Technology in Poultry Meat Industry: A Vision to 2020. Poultry Research Priorities to 2020 Proceedings *of National Seminar (November 2-3). Central Avian Research Institute* (Indian Council of Agricultural Research). Izatnagar-243 122 (U.P.), India.

Ross, S.A., Srinivas, P.R., Clifford, A.J., Lee, S.C., Philbert, M.A., and Hettich, R.L. (2004): New technologies for nutrition research. *Journals of Nutrition,* **134**: 681-685.

Scott, N.R., (2005): Nanotechnology and Animal health. *Revised scienceof technology of International Epizootic,* **24**: 425. DOI:10.1016/j.jtbi.2008.

Seleem, M. N., Jain, N., Pothayee, N., Ranjan, A., Rffle, J. S., and Sriragana, N. (2009): Targeting *Brucella melitensis* with polymeric nanoparticles containing streptomycin and doxycycline. *FEMS Microbialogy Letters,* **294**: 24–31.

Semih, O., and Buket, Yalcin. (2008): Smart food packaging. Elektroniczne czasopismo naukowe z dziedziny logistyki, **4**(3): 4. http://www.logforum.net . Accessed on March, 29, 2017.

Si, D.Y., Liang, W., Sun, D.Y., Cheng, F.T., and Liu, C.X. (2007): Nanoscale devices for veterinary technology: Trends and future prospective. *Asian Journal of Pharmacodynamics and Pharmacokinetics,* **7**(2): 83. DOI: 10.1007/s11671-010-9597-y

Strijkers, G.J., Mulder, W.J., Vanheeswijk, R.B., Frederik, P.M., Bomans, P., Magusin, P.C.; and Nicolay, K. (2005): Relaxivity of liposomal paramagnetic MRI contrast agents, *MAGMA,* **18**: 186. DOI: 10.1007/s10334-005-0111-y

Suga, K., Mikawa, M., Ogasawara, N., Okazaki, H., and Matsunaga, N. (2001): Potential of Gd- DTPA-mannan liposome particles as a pulmonary perfusion MRI contrast agent: an initial animal study. *Investigate Radiology,* **36**:130.

Suh, W.H., Suslick, K.S., Slucky.G. D., and Suh, Y.H. (2009): Nanotechnology, nanotoxicology, and neuroscience. *Progress Neurobiology.* **87**:133–170.

Svenson, S., Tomalia, D.A. (2005): Dendrimers in biomedical applications – reflections on the field. *Advance Drug Delivery Revised,* **57**: 2106– 2129.

Taylor, T.M., Davidson, P.M., Bruce, B.D., and Weiss, J. (2005): Liposomal nanocapsules in food science and agriculture. *Critical Revised Food Science Nutrition,* **45**: 1-19

Tiwari, A., (2011): Advanced materials world congress, Sweden. *Advance materials letters*, **2**(6):377. DOI:10.5185/amlett.2011.1200.

Tiwari, A., and Dhakate, S.R. (2009): BIOPOLYMER NANOCOMPOSITES *.International Journal of Biological Macromolecules*, **44**: 480. DOI: 10.1016/j.ijbiomac.2009.03.002

Troncarelli, M.Z., Brandão, H.M., Gern, J.C., Guimarães, A.S., Langoni, H., Gern, J.C., Bernardes, F. (2012) Published in: Mastite bovina sob nanocontrole: a própolis nanoestruturada como nova perspectiva de tratamento para rebanhosleiteiros orgânicos. Vet. Zootec., v.20, Edição Comemorativa, jun 2013. Available in http://www.fmvz.unesp.br/rvz/index.php/rvz/article/view/657. Accessed on march, 29, 2017.

Verma, O.P., R. Kumar, A. Kumar and S. Chand, (2012):.Assisted reproductive techniques in farm animal:from artificial insemination to Nanobiotechnology.*Vet World*, **5**: 301-310.

Wei, Q., Xu, C., Wei, Q., Du, B., Li, R., Zhang, T., Wu, D., and Dai, W. (2010): Nanoscale device for veterinary technology: Trends and future prospective. *Advance Material Letters*, **1**(3): 217. DOI: 10.5185/amlett.2010.3104.

Weibel, M.I., J.M. Badano and I. Rintoul, (2014): Technological evolution of hormone deliverysystems for estrous synchronization in cattle. *International Journal of Livestock Research*, **4**: 20-40.

You, C.C., Miranda, O.R., Gider, B., Ghosh, P.S., Kim, I.B., Erdogan, B.; Krovi, S.A., Bunz, U.H.F., and Rotello, V.M. (2007): Detection and identification of proteins using nanoparticle-fluorescent polymer 'chemical nose' sensors, *Nature Nanotechnololgy*. **2**: 318. DOI: 10.1038/nnano.2007.99

Zampoli, M., Troncarelli,H., Mello Brandao ,J. Carine Gern,A. Sá Guimarães and H. Langoni. (2008): The Relevance for Food Safety of Applications of Nanotechnology in the Food and Feed Industries. ISBN 1-90Pp. 4465-59588p.

Zhang, L., GU, F. X., Chan, J., M, Wang, A., Z, Langer, R., S, Farokhzad, O., C. (2008): Nanoparticles in medicine: therapeutic applications and developments. *Clinical PharmacololgyTherapeutics*. **83**:761-769.

Zhang, L., Pornpattananangkul, D., and Hung, C.M. (2010): Development of Nanoparticles for Antimicrobial Drug Delivery. *Current Medicinal Chemistry*, 17: 585-594

Zhao, H., Zhang, Z., Zhao, Z., Yu, R., Wan, Y., Lan, M. (2011): Nanoscale devices for veterinar technology: Trends. Advance Material Letters, 2(3):172. DOI:10.5185/amlett.2011.1210

Zheng, J., Perkins, G., Kirilova, A., Allen, C., Jaffray DA .(2006): Multimodal contrast agent for combined computed tomography and magnetic resonance imaging applications. *Invest Radiol*, **41**: 339-348.